THE MIND DIET PLAN FOR BEGINNERS

Eating for Brain Health: A Nutrition Plan for Preventing and Managing Alzheimer's and Dementia

DR JULIA R. ARTHUR

DR JULIA R. ARTHUR

TABLE OF CONTENTS

INTRODUCTION

Nicole is a sixty-year-old woman who had been suffering from Alzheimer's for the past few years. She had been struggling to remember even the simplest things, such as her own name or her family members. She had been to numerous doctors and specialists who had all recommended different treatments, but none of them had any success.

One day, Nicole stumbled across this book that promised a revolutionary new diet plan that could help reverse the effects of Alzheimer's. At first, she was skeptical, but she decided to give it a try. She followed the diet plan for several weeks, and gradually, she began to notice positive changes.

Nicole's memory started to improve, and she was able to recall more and more details every day. She started to recognize her family members more and more, and she could even complete simple tasks that she had once found difficult.

After some months of following the diet plan, Nicole was amazed to find that she had completely reversed her Alzheimer's! She was able to remember even the most obscure details, and she could carry on conversations with ease.

Nicole was overjoyed to have her life back, and she was so grateful to have found the right diet plan in the book. She was living proof that it was possible to reverse the effects of Alzheimer's, and she was determined to spread the word about this revolutionary diet plan to others.

Alzheimer's disease and dementia are two of the most common causes of cognitive decline in older adults. Alzheimer's disease is a progressive neurological disorder that slowly destroys memory and other cognitive functions. Dementia is an umbrella term used to describe a wide range of symptoms that occur when the brain is impaired by disease or injury. While Alzheimer's disease is the most common cause of dementia, there are many other causes.

Alzheimer's disease is characterized by the buildup of two proteins in the brain – amyloid and tau. As these proteins accumulate, they form plaques and tangles that damage and destroy the nerve cells. This damage impairs the brain's ability to function normally and leads to memory loss, confusion, and behavioral changes.

Dementia is a general term used to describe the decline in cognitive function caused by a variety of conditions, including Alzheimer's disease, stroke, and Parkinson's disease. It can affect memory, attention, language, judgment, and problem-solving skills. Symptoms vary depending on the cause, but can include difficulty concentrating, apathy, confusion, and difficulty managing daily tasks.

Although Alzheimer's disease and dementia are both serious, progressive conditions, there are treatments and strategies that can help people with these conditions. These include medications, lifestyle changes, diets, and support from family and friends. It is also important to remember that, while these conditions cannot be cured, they can be managed. With the right care and support, people with Alzheimer's disease and dementia can live meaningful lives.

CHAPTER 1

Understanding Alzheimer's and Dementia

Alzheimer's and Dementia are two of the most common types of age-related dementia, which is a general term used to describe a decline in cognitive function. Alzheimer's is a specific form of dementia, whereas Dementia encompasses a range of different conditions that affect memory, thinking, behavior and social abilities.

Alzheimer's is a progressive, degenerative disease that affects the brain's ability to store and recall information. It is the most common form of age-related dementia, and its symptoms usually appear in people aged over 65 years. The most common symptoms of Alzheimer's are memory loss, difficulty thinking or problem-solving, difficulty with language, difficulty with motor skills, and changes in behavior.

Dementia, unlike Alzheimer's, can be caused by several different conditions. These include stroke, Parkinson's disease, Huntington's disease, and HIV/AIDS. The symptoms of dementia vary depending on the cause, but generally include memory loss, difficulty thinking and problem-solving, difficulty with language, difficulty with motor skills, and changes in behavior.

The causes of both Alzheimer's and Dementia are largely unknown but researchers are working to improve our understanding. Risk factors for Alzheimer's and Dementia include age, family history, lifestyle, and medical conditions.

There is currently no cure for either Alzheimer's or Dementia, but treatments are available to help manage symptoms and slow the progression of the disease.

It is important to be aware of the symptoms of Alzheimer's and Dementia, as early diagnosis and intervention can help to delay the progression of the disease and improve the quality of life for those affected. If you or someone you know is experiencing any of the symptoms of Alzheimer's or Dementia, it is important to seek medical advice.

There are also a range of support services available to those living with Alzheimer's and Dementia, including support groups, education programs and access to specialized care.

It is important to remember that those living with Alzheimer's and Dementia are still capable of living meaningful lives, and that they should be treated with respect and understanding.

Understanding Alzheimer's and Dementia can help to reduce the stigma associated with these conditions, and can help to ensure that those living with them receive the care and support they need.

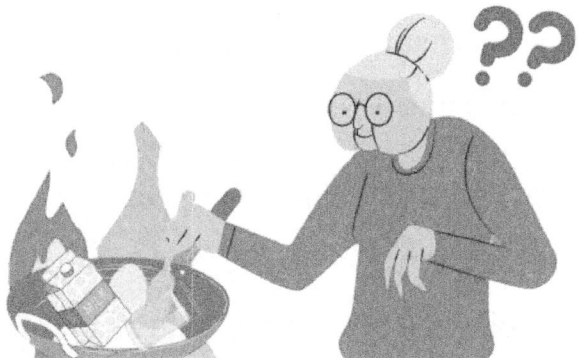

Risk Factors and Prevention Tips

Alzheimer's and dementia are two of the most common forms of cognitive decline that can occur in older adults. Risk factors for Alzheimer's and dementia include age, genetics, lifestyle, and medical conditions.

Age: As you age, your risk for dementia increases. The greatest risk for dementia is found in those 80 years of age or older.

Genetics: Having a family history of Alzheimer's or dementia increases your risk for developing the condition.

Lifestyle: Poor diet, lack of physical activity, and excessive alcohol consumption are all lifestyle choices that could increase your risk for Alzheimer's and dementia.

Medical Conditions: Diabetes, stroke, high blood pressure, and heart disease can all increase your risk for dementia.

There are steps you can take to help reduce your risk of developing Alzheimer's and dementia. Eating a healthy diet, exercising regularly, and getting plenty of sleep are all important components of reducing your risk. Additionally, maintaining a strong social network and engaging in stimulating activities can also help reduce your risk.

Despite the known risk factors, it is still not possible to predict who will develop Alzheimer's or dementia. While it is important to be aware of the risk factors, it is also important to remember that you can still lead a full and healthy life regardless of your risk.

By taking steps to reduce your risk, staying engaged in activities that promote cognitive health, and seeking medical attention if you have any concerns, you can help reduce your chances of developing Alzheimer's or dementia.

If your doctor diagnoses you with Alzheimer's or dementia, it is important to remember that there are still ways to manage your condition and maintain a high quality of life.

PREVENTIVE TIPS

1. Exercise regularly: Exercise helps keep your body and mind healthy. Regular physical activity can help improve brain health and reduce the risk of cognitive decline, including dementia.

2. Eat a healthy diet: Eating a healthy diet with plenty of fruits, vegetables, and whole grains can help reduce your risk of cognitive decline and dementia.

3. Stay socially active: Social interaction is important for maintaining cognitive health. Participating in activities like book clubs, classes, or volunteering can help keep your brain active and engaged.

4. Stay mentally active: Mental activities like reading, crosswords, and puzzles can help keep your brain active and increase your cognitive reserve.

5. Get enough sleep: Getting enough quality sleep is important for cognitive health. Research suggests that people who sleep fewer than six hours a night are at higher risk of dementia.

6. Quit smoking: Quitting smoking can help reduce your risk of cognitive decline and dementia.

7. Manage your stress: Stress can have a negative impact on your brain, so it's important to find ways to manage it.

8. Take vitamins and supplements: Certain vitamins and supplements have been linked to cognitive health.

9. Get regular check-ups: Regular check-ups can help you detect and diagnose any medical conditions that could increase your risk of dementia.

10. Challenge your brain: Challenging your brain with activities like yoga, meditation, and learning a new language can help keep your brain healthy and reduce your risk of dementia.

11. Stay organized: Organization can help reduce stress and keep your brain healthy.

12. Take care of your heart health: Heart health is linked to brain health, so it's important to take steps to keep your heart healthy.

13. Stay connected: Connecting with friends and family can help reduce stress and keep your brain active.

14. Monitor your medications: Certain medications can increase your risk of dementia, so it's important to talk to your doctor about any medications you're taking.

15. Participate in social activities: Participating in social activities like attending a class or joining a club can help keep your brain active.

Natural Remedies and Therapies

Alzheimer's and dementia are progressive neurological diseases that can cause a wide range of physical and cognitive symptoms. While there is currently no known cure for these conditions, there are a number of natural remedies that may help improve symptoms and slow the progression of the disease.

1. Exercise: Exercise can help to improve cognitive function and reduce the risk of developing dementia. Regular physical activity can improve circulation, reduce stress, and stimulate the production of neurotransmitters that are important for memory and cognitive functioning.

2. Cognitive Training: Cognitive training is also known as brain games and can help to improve mental function in people with Alzheimer's and dementia. Cognitive training involves activities such as crosswords and puzzles that help to strengthen the connections between the brain cells and improve the ability to recall memories.

3. Omega-3 Fatty Acids: Omega-3 fatty acids have been found to have neuroprotective effects and may help to reduce the risk of Alzheimer's and dementia. They can be found in foods such as salmon, mackerel, and sardines as well as in supplement form.

4. Turmeric: Turmeric is a spice that has been used in traditional Indian medicine for centuries. It contains an active ingredient called curcumin which has been found to have anti-inflammatory and antioxidant properties. Studies have suggested that it may help to improve cognitive function in people with Alzheimer's and dementia.

5. Ginkgo Biloba: Ginkgo biloba is an herb that has been used traditionally to improve memory and cognitive function. Studies have suggested that it may help to reduce the risk of cognitive decline in people with Alzheimer's and dementia.

6. Acupuncture: Acupuncture is a traditional Chinese medicine practice that involves the insertion of needles into specific points in the body. Studies have suggested that it may help to improve cognitive function in people with Alzheimer's and dementia.

7. Vitamins and Minerals: Vitamins and minerals such as B vitamins, vitamin D, and magnesium have been found to have neuroprotective effects and may help to reduce the risk of cognitive decline in people with Alzheimer's and dementia.

Though these natural remedies may help to improve symptoms and slow the progression of the disease, it is important to note that they should not be used as a substitute for medical advice or treatment. It is important to speak with a healthcare professional before starting any new natural remedy.

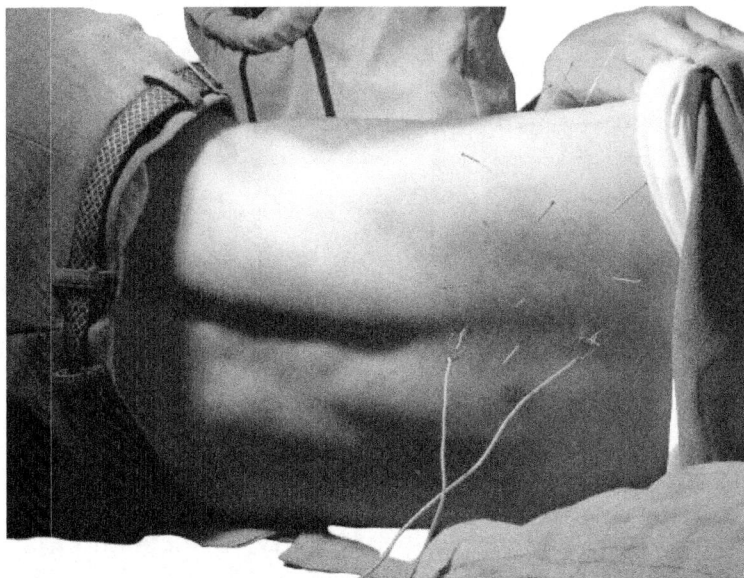

CHAPTER 2

Exercises to Reverse Alzheimer and Dementia

Memory exercises: Memory exercises can help individuals with Alzheimer's disease or dementia practice recalling information and improve their memory skills. Examples of memory exercises include:

1. Remembering a list of items (e.g., groceries or errands)
2. Recalling the name of a person after being introduced
3. Repeating a sequence of numbers or letters
4. Playing memory games (e.g., Concentration or Memory Match)

Language and communication exercises: Language and communication exercises can help individuals with Alzheimer's disease or dementia practice their verbal and written communication skills. Examples of language and communication exercises include:

1. Reading aloud from a book or newspaper
2. Having conversations with a partner or caregiver
3. Sending messages to loved ones
4. Playing word games (e.g., Scrabble or Banana grams)

Physical exercises: Physical exercises can help individuals with Alzheimer's disease or dementia maintain their physical strength and mobility. Examples of physical exercises include:

1. Going for a walk or bike ride
2. Doing gentle stretches or yoga poses
3. Participating in chair exercises (e.g., seated leg lifts or arm curls)
4. Dancing to music

Cognitive exercises: Cognitive exercises can help individuals with Alzheimer's disease or dementia practice their problem-solving and critical thinking skills. Examples of cognitive exercises include:

1. Doing crossword puzzles or Sudoku
2. Playing strategy games (e.g., chess or Go)
3. Doing jigsaw puzzles
4. Solving riddles or brainteasers

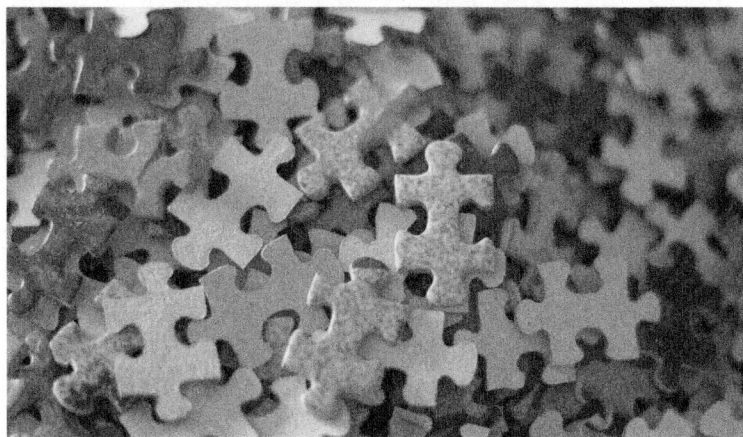

Lifestyle Changes to Combat Cognitive Decline

There are several lifestyle changes that individuals can make to help combat cognitive decline:

Exercise regularly: Regular physical activity has been shown to improve brain health and cognitive function. Aim for at least 150 minutes of moderate-intensity exercise per week, such as brisk walking, swimming, or cycling.

Eat a healthy diet: A healthy diet rich in fruits, vegetables, and healthy fats (such as those found in nuts, seeds, and avocados) has been linked to better cognitive function. Avoid processed and sugary foods, as they have been linked to cognitive decline.

Get enough sleep: Adequate sleep is important for brain health and cognitive function. Aim for 7-9 hours of sleep per night.

Stay mentally active: Engaging in activities that challenge the brain, such as reading, doing crossword puzzles, or learning a new skill, can help keep the brain active and may help slow cognitive decline.

Stay socially active: Social connections and activities have been linked to better cognitive function. Make an effort to stay connected with friends and family, and participate in social activities that you enjoy.

Reduce stress: Chronic stress has been linked to cognitive decline. Practice stress-reduction techniques such as meditation, yoga, or deep breathing to help manage stress.

Avoid risky behaviors: Avoiding risky behaviors such as smoking and excessive alcohol consumption can help protect against cognitive decline.

Coping with Caregiving

Caregiving for a loved one with Alzheimer's disease or dementia can be a challenging and demanding role. Here are some tips for coping with caregiving:

Take care of yourself: It's important to prioritize your own physical and emotional well-being while caregiving. Make sure to eat well, get enough rest, and participate in activities that you enjoy. It's also important to seek support from others, such as friends, family, or a support group.

Set boundaries: Caregiving can be all-consuming, so it's important to set boundaries and make time for yourself. This can help prevent burnout and ensure that you have the energy and resources to continue caring for your loved one.

Seek out resources: There are many resources available to caregivers of individuals with Alzheimer's disease or dementia, such as respite care, in-home support, and support groups. Don't be afraid to ask for help or to utilize these resources.

Communicate with your loved one: Individuals with Alzheimer's disease or dementia may have difficulty expressing their needs and feelings. It's important to try to communicate with your loved one in a way that is respectful and understanding. This may involve using nonverbal cues, simplifying language, and being patient.

Stay organized: Caregiving can be overwhelming, so it's important to stay organized and create a care plan that works for you and your loved one. This can include tasks such as scheduling doctor's appointments, organizing medication, and making arrangements for respite care.

Find ways to manage stress: Caregiving can be stressful, so it's important to find ways to manage stress and take care of your own well-being. This can include practicing relaxation techniques, getting regular exercise, or seeking support from friends and family.

It's important to remember that caregiving is a challenging but rewarding role. Seeking out resources and support can help make the caregiving journey easier.

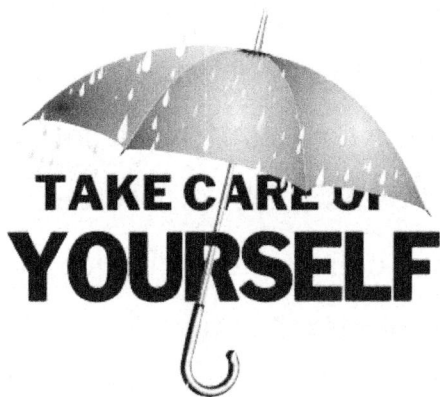

TAKE CARE OF
YOURSELF

Alzheimer's Meal Plan

Day 1

Breakfast: Scrambled eggs with whole grain toast and fruit

Snack: Greek yogurt with berries and nuts

Lunch: Turkey and avocado wrap with whole grain crackers and fruit

Snack: Apple slices with almond butter

Dinner: Grilled chicken with roasted vegetables and quinoa

Day 2

Breakfast: Oatmeal with nuts, dried fruit, and a splash of almond milk

Snack: Hard-boiled egg with whole grain crackers

Lunch: Whole grain pita stuffed with hummus, roasted vegetables, and grilled chicken

Snack: Carrot sticks with hummus

Dinner: Slow cooker lentil soup with a side of whole grain bread

Day 3

Breakfast: Whole grain toast with almond butter and sliced banana

Snack: Greek yogurt with berries and nuts

Lunch: Whole grain pasta with roasted vegetables and a homemade tomato sauce

Snack: Apple slices with peanut butter

Dinner: Grilled salmon with roasted vegetables and quinoa

Day 4

Breakfast: Smoothie made with banana, spinach, protein powder, and almond milk

Snack: Hard-boiled egg with whole grain crackers

Lunch: Quinoa and black bean salad with avocado, cherry tomatoes, and lemon vinaigrette

Snack: Carrot sticks with hummus

Dinner: Baked sweet potato topped with black beans, salsa, and guacamole

Day 5

Breakfast: Scrambled eggs with spinach and whole grain toast

Snack: Greek yogurt with berries and nuts

Lunch: Whole grain crackers with hummus and veggies

Snack: Apple slices with almond butter

Dinner: Grilled chicken with roasted broccoli and quinoa

Day 6

Breakfast: Overnight oats with chia seeds, berries, and almond milk

Snack: Hard-boiled egg with whole grain crackers

Lunch: Whole grain pita stuffed with falafel, tzatziki sauce, and veggies

Snack: Carrot sticks with hummus

Dinner: Baked salmon with roasted asparagus and quinoa

DAY 7

Breakfast: Greek yogurt with nuts, berries, and a drizzle of honey

Snack: Apple slices with peanut butter

Lunch: Whole grain pasta with roasted vegetables and a homemade tomato sauce

Snack: Greek yogurt with berries and nuts

Dinner: Slow cooker black bean and sweet potato chili with a side of cornbread

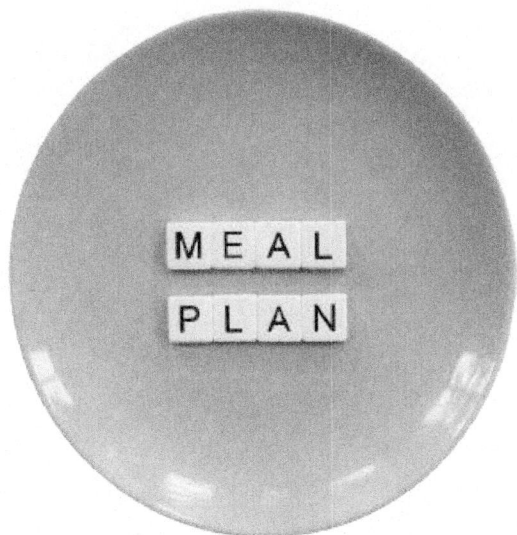

CHAPTER 3

Alzheimer and Dementia Recipes

Breakfast

Banana Oatmeal Porridge

Ingredients:

- ½ cup oatmeal

- 2 ripe bananas

- 1 cup of milk

- 2 tbsp of honey

- 1 tsp of ground cinnamon

- 2 tbsp of walnuts

- 2 tbsp of raisins

Instructions:

1. Place the oatmeal and milk in a pot over medium heat.

2. Cook for 5 minutes, stirring constantly.

3. Mash the bananas and add them to the pot.

4. Cook for an additional 2 minutes, stirring constantly.

5. Stir in the honey and cinnamon.

6. Cook until the porridge is the desired consistency.

7. Garnish with the walnuts and raisins.

Time: 10 minutes

Chia Seed Pudding

Ingredients:

- ½ cup chia seeds

- 2 cups of milk

- 2 tbsp of honey

- 1 tsp of ground cinnamon

- 2 tbsp of dried cranberries

- 2 tbsp of sliced almonds

Instructions:

1. Place the chia seeds, milk, and honey in a bowl and mix until combined.

2. Cover and refrigerate overnight.

3. In the morning, stir in the cinnamon.

4. Divide the pudding among 4 bowls.

5. Top with the cranberries and almonds.

Time: 10 minutes (plus overnight soaking time)

Egg Muffins

Ingredients:

- 6 eggs

- ½ cup of diced bell pepper

- ½ cup of diced onion

- ½ cup of shredded cheese

- Salt and pepper to taste

Instructions:

1. Preheat oven to 375°F.

2. Grease a muffin tin with cooking spray.

3. In a bowl, whisk together the eggs, bell pepper, onion, cheese, and salt and pepper.

4. Divide the mixture among the muffin tin cups.

5. Bake for 15 minutes.

Time: 20 minutes

Savory Oatmeal Bowl

Ingredients:

- ½ cup oatmeal

- 2 cups of water

- 1 tbsp of olive oil

- ½ cup of diced bell pepper

- ½ cup of diced onion

- ½ cup of shredded cheese

- Salt and pepper to taste

Instructions:

1. Place the oatmeal and water in a pot over medium heat.

2. Cook for 5 minutes, stirring constantly.

3. Heat the olive oil in a skillet over medium heat.

4. Add the bell pepper and onion and cook for 5 minutes.

5. Stir the bell pepper and onion into the oatmeal.

6. Stir in the cheese and season with salt and pepper.

Time: 10 minutes

Baked Apples

Ingredients:

- 4 apples, cored and sliced

- 2 tbsp of butter, melted

- 2 tbsp of brown sugar

- 2 tbsp of raisins

- 1 tsp of ground cinnamon

- 2 tbsp of chopped walnuts

Instructions:

1. Preheat oven to 375°F.

2. Grease a baking dish with cooking spray.

3. Place the apples in the baking dish.

4. Drizzle with the melted butter and sprinkle with the brown sugar, raisins, cinnamon, and walnuts.

5. Bake for 15 minutes.

Time: 20 minutes

Smoothie Bowl

Ingredients:

- 2 cups of frozen mixed berries

- 1 banana

- 1 cup of milk

- 1 tsp of ground flaxseed

- 2 tbsp of shredded coconut

- 2 tbsp of sliced almonds

Instructions:

1. Place the frozen berries, banana, and milk in a blender and blend until smooth.

2. Pour the smoothie into a bowl.

3. Sprinkle with the flaxseed, coconut, and almonds.

Time: 5 minutes

Veggie Omelette

Ingredients:

- 4 eggs

- ½ cup of diced bell pepper

- ½ cup of diced onion

- ½ cup of diced mushrooms

- Salt and pepper to taste

Instructions:

1. Heat a skillet over medium heat.

2. In a bowl, whisk together the eggs, bell pepper, onion, mushrooms, and salt and pepper.

3. Pour the mixture into the skillet and cook for 5 minutes.

4. Flip the omelette and cook for an additional 5 minutes.

Time: 10 minutes

Baked Oatmeal

Ingredients:

- 2 cups of oats

- 2 cups of milk

- 2 ripe bananas

- 2 tbsp of honey

- 1 tsp of ground cinnamon

- 2 tbsp of raisins

- 2 tbsp of chopped walnuts

Instructions:

1. Preheat the oven to 375°F.

2. Grease a baking dish with cooking spray.

3. Place the oats and milk in the baking dish and stir to combine.

4. Mash the bananas and spread over the oat mixture.

5. Drizzle with the honey and sprinkle with the cinnamon, raisins, and walnuts.

6. Bake for 15 minutes.

Time: 20 minutes

Avocado Toast

Ingredients:

- 2 slices of whole grain bread

- 1 ripe avocado

- 2 tbsp of olive oil

- 1 tsp of lemon juice

- Salt and pepper to taste

Instructions:

1. Toast the bread.

2. Mash the avocado and spread on the toast.

3. Drizzle with the olive oil and lemon juice and season with salt and pepper.

Time: 5 minutes

Yogurt Parfait

Ingredients:

- 1 cup of plain yogurt

- 2 tbsp of honey

- 2 tbsp of granola

- 2 tbsp of dried cran

- 2 tbsp of sliced almonds

Instructions:

1. Place the yogurt in a bowl.

2. Drizzle with the honey.

3. Top with the granola, cranberries, and almonds.

Time: 5 minutes

LUNCH

Baked Salmon with Asparagus and Tomatoes

Ingredients: 4 salmon fillets, 2 tablespoons olive oil, 1 teaspoon ground black pepper, 1 teaspoon garlic powder, 2 bunches asparagus, 3 tomatoes, 1 tablespoon chopped fresh basil.

Cooking Instructions: Preheat oven to 375 degrees F (190 degrees C). Grease a baking dish with olive oil. Place salmon fillets in the dish. Drizzle with olive oil and sprinkle with black pepper and garlic powder. Arrange asparagus and tomatoes around the salmon. Bake in preheated oven for 20 minutes, or until fish flakes easily with a fork. Sprinkle with basil before serving.

Prep Time: 10 minutes

Cook Time: 20 minutes

Baked Chicken with Spinach and Oranges

Ingredients: 4 boneless, skinless chicken breasts, 2 tablespoons olive oil, 2 cloves garlic, minced, 4 cups fresh spinach, 2 oranges, peeled and sliced, 1 teaspoon ground black pepper.

Cooking Instructions: Preheat oven to 375 degrees F (190 degrees C). Grease a baking dish with olive oil. Place chicken breasts in the baking dish. Drizzle with olive oil and sprinkle with garlic. Top with spinach, oranges, and pepper. Bake in preheated oven for 25 minutes, or until chicken is cooked through.

Prep Time: 10 minutes

Cook Time: 25 minutes

Quinoa with Broccoli and Mushrooms

Ingredients: 1 cup quinoa, 2 cups vegetable broth, 2 tablespoons olive oil, 1 clove garlic, minced, 1 head broccoli, chopped, 8 ounces mushrooms, sliced, 1 teaspoon ground black pepper.

Cooking Instructions: Heat olive oil in a large saucepan over medium heat. Add garlic and cook for 1 minute. Add quinoa and vegetable broth and bring to a boil. Reduce heat to low, cover and simmer for 15 minutes, or until liquid is absorbed. Stir in broccoli and mushrooms. Simmer for 10 minutes, or until vegetables are tender. Season with pepper.

Prep Time: 10 minutes

Cook Time: 25 minutes

Vegetable Stir-Fry with Rice

Ingredients: 2 tablespoons olive oil, 1 onion, chopped, 2 cloves garlic, minced, 1 red bell pepper, chopped, 1 yellow bell pepper, chopped, 2 carrots, sliced, 1 head broccoli, chopped, 2 cups cooked white rice, 1 teaspoon ground black pepper.

Cooking Instructions: Heat olive oil in a large skillet over medium-high heat. Add onion and garlic and cook for 2 minutes. Add bell peppers, carrots, and broccoli and cook for 5 minutes, stirring occasionally. Stir in cooked rice and season with black pepper. Cook for 5 minutes, stirring occasionally.

Prep Time: 10 minutes

Cook Time: 12 minutes

Baked Tofu with Broccoli and Rice

Ingredients: 1 package extra-firm tofu, drained and cubed, 2 tablespoons olive oil, 2 cloves garlic, minced, 1 head broccoli, chopped, 2 cups cooked white rice, 1 teaspoon ground black pepper.

Cooking Instructions: Preheat oven to 375 degrees F (190 degrees C). Grease a baking dish with olive oil. Place tofu cubes in the dish. Drizzle with olive oil and sprinkle with garlic. Top with broccoli and rice. Bake in preheated oven for 25 minutes, or until tofu is golden brown. Sprinkle with pepper before serving.

Prep Time: 10 minutes

Cook Time: 25 minutes

Roasted Vegetables with Brown Rice

Ingredients: 2 tablespoons olive oil, 1 onion, chopped, 2 cloves garlic, minced, 1 head broccoli, chopped, 2 carrots, sliced, 1 red bell pepper, chopped, 2 cups cooked brown rice, 1 teaspoon ground black pepper.

Cooking Instructions: Preheat oven to 375 degrees F (190 degrees C). Grease a baking dish with olive oil. Place onion, garlic, broccoli, carrots, and bell pepper in the dish. Drizzle with olive oil and sprinkle with black pepper. Bake in preheated oven for 25 minutes, or until vegetables are tender. Serve over cooked brown rice.

Prep Time: 10 minutes

Cook Time: 25 minutes

Baked Zucchini with Tomatoes and Rice

Ingredients: 2 zucchinis, sliced, 2 tablespoons olive oil, 2 cloves garlic, minced, 2 tomatoes, chopped, 2 cups cooked white rice, 1 teaspoon ground black pepper.

Cooking Instructions: Preheat oven to 375 degrees F (190 degrees C). Grease a baking dish with olive oil. Place zucchini in the dish. Drizzle with olive oil and sprinkle with garlic. Top with tomatoes. Bake in preheated oven for 20 minutes, or until zucchini is tender. Serve over cooked rice and sprinkle with pepper before serving.

Prep Time: 10 minutes

Cook Time: 20 minutes

Lentil Soup with Spinach and Carrots

Ingredients: 2 tablespoons olive oil, 1 onion, chopped, 2 cloves garlic, minced, 2 carrots, chopped, 2 cups cooked lentils, 4 cups vegetable broth, 2 cups fresh spinach, 1 teaspoon ground black pepper.

Cooking Instructions: Heat olive oil in a large saucepan over medium heat. Add onion and garlic and cook for 2 minutes. Add carrots and lentils and cook for 3 minutes. Stir in vegetable broth and bring to a boil. Reduce heat to low and simmer for 20 minutes. Stir in spinach and season with pepper. Simmer for 5 minutes, or until spinach is wilted.

Prep Time: 10 minutes

Cook Time: 30 minutes

Vegetable Fried Rice

Ingredients: 2 tablespoons olive oil, 1 onion, chopped, 2 cloves garlic, minced, 1 head broccoli, chopped, 2 carrots, sliced, 2 cups cooked white rice, 2 tablespoons soy sauce, 1 teaspoon ground black pepper.

Cooking Instructions: Heat olive oil in a large skillet over medium-high heat. Add onion and garlic and cook for 2 minutes. Add broccoli and carrots and cook for 5 minutes, stirring occasionally. Stir in cooked rice, soy sauce, and pepper. Cook for 5 minutes, stirring occasionally.

Prep Time: 10 minutes

Cook Time: 12 minutes

Baked Cod with Asparagus and Potatoes

Ingredients: 4 cod fillets, 2 tablespoons olive oil, 1 teaspoon ground black pepper, 2 cloves garlic, minced, 4 potatoes, chopped, 2 bunches asparagus, 1 teaspoon dried oregano.

Cooking Instructions: Preheat oven to 375 degrees F (190 degrees C). Grease a baking dish with olive oil. Place cod fillets in the dish. Drizzle with olive oil and sprinkle with black pepper and garlic. Arrange potatoes and asparagus around the cod. Sprinkle with oregano. Bake in preheated oven for 20 minutes, or until fish flakes easily with a fork.

Prep Time: 10 minutes

Cook Time: 20 minutes

DINNER

Baked Salmon with Asparagus and Sweet Potatoes

Preparation time: 10 minutes, Cooking time: 30 minutes

Ingredients:

- 2 6-ounce salmon filets

- 1 pound asparagus

- 2 medium sweet potatoes, cubed

- 2 tablespoons olive oil

- Salt and pepper to taste

Instructions:

1. Preheat oven to 375 degrees F.

2. Place sweet potatoes in a baking dish, drizzle with olive oil, and season with salt and pepper. Bake in the preheated oven for 15 minutes.

3. Meanwhile, rinse the asparagus and cut into 1-inch pieces.

4. After the sweet potatoes have been baking for 15 minutes, add the asparagus to the baking dish.

5. Place the salmon filets on top of the asparagus and season with salt and pepper.

6. Bake in the preheated oven for an additional 15 minutes or until the salmon is cooked through and the vegetables are tender.

Oven-Baked Chicken and Rice

Preparation time: 10 minutes, Cooking time: 45 minutes

Ingredients:

- 2 boneless, skinless chicken breasts

- 1 cup uncooked white rice

- 1 cup chicken broth

- 1 cup sliced mushrooms

- 1 teaspoon olive oil

- Salt and pepper to taste

Instructions:

1. Preheat oven to 350 degrees F.

2. Place chicken breasts in a baking dish.

3. In a separate bowl, combine the rice, chicken broth, mushrooms, olive oil, and salt and pepper. Pour the mixture over the chicken.

4. Cover with foil and bake in the preheated oven for 30 minutes.

5. Remove the foil and bake for an additional 15 minutes or until the chicken is cooked through and the rice is tender.

Spinach and Ricotta Stuffed Shells

Preparation time: 10 minutes, Cooking time: 30 minutes

Ingredients:

- 12 jumbo pasta shells

- 2 cups ricotta cheese

- 1 10-ounce package frozen chopped spinach, thawed and drained

- 1 cup shredded mozzarella cheese

- 1/4 cup grated Parmesan cheese

- 1 teaspoon garlic powder

- Salt and pepper to taste

- 1 24-ounce jar of your favorite marinara sauce

Instructions:

1. Preheat oven to 350 degrees F.

2. Cook pasta shells in boiling salted water for 8 minutes, or until al dente. Drain and set aside.

3. In a medium bowl, combine the ricotta cheese, spinach, mozzarella cheese, Parmesan cheese, garlic powder, and salt and pepper.

4. Stuff the cooked shells with the ricotta cheese mixture and place in a 9x13-inch baking dish.

5. Pour the marinara sauce over the shells and bake in the preheated oven for 20 minutes.

Easy Baked Fish

Preparation time: 10 minutes, Cooking time: 20 minutes

Ingredients:

- 2 6-ounce white fish fillets (cod, haddock, or tilapia)

- 2 tablespoons butter

- 1 tablespoon lemon juice

- 1/4 cup dry white wine

- 1/4 teaspoon garlic powder

- Salt and pepper to taste

- 2 tablespoons minced fresh parsley

Instructions:

1. Preheat oven to 350 degrees F.

2. Place fish in a baking dish.

3. In a small bowl, combine the butter, lemon juice, white wine, garlic powder, salt, and pepper. Pour the mixture over the fish.

4. Bake in the preheated oven for 20 minutes or until the fish is cooked through.

5. Garnish with minced parsley before serving.

Baked Vegetarian Lasagna

Preparation time: 10 minutes, Cooking time: 45 minutes

Ingredients:

- 1 16-ounce container ricotta cheese

- 1/2 cup grated Parmesan cheese

- 1 10-ounce package frozen chopped spinach, thawed and drained

- 1 24-ounce jar of your favorite marinara sauce

- 1/2 teaspoon garlic powder

- 12 uncooked lasagna noodles

- 2 cups shredded mozzarella cheese

Instructions:

1. Preheat oven to 375 degrees F.

2. In a medium bowl, combine the ricotta cheese, Parmesan cheese, spinach, garlic powder, and salt and pepper.

3. Spread 1/4 cup of marinara sauce in the bottom of a 9x13-inch baking dish.

4. Layer 4 uncooked lasagna noodles on top of the sauce.

5. Spread half of the ricotta cheese mixture on top of the noodles.

6. Top with 1/4 cup of marinara sauce and 1 cup of mozzarella cheese.

7. Layer with 4 more noodles and the remaining ricotta cheese mixture.

8. Top with 1/4 cup marinara sauce and 1 cup mozzarella cheese.

9. Layer with 4 more noodles and the remaining marinara sauce.

10. Sprinkle with remaining mozzarella cheese.

11. Cover with foil and bake in the preheated oven for 30 minutes.

12. Remove the foil and bake for an additional 15 minutes or until the cheese is melted and bubbly.

Creamy Chicken and Rice Soup

Preparation time: 10 minutes, Cooking time: 25 minutes

Ingredients:

- 2 tablespoons butter

- 1/2 cup diced onion

- 1/2 cup diced celery

- 1/2 cup diced carrots

- 1 cup diced cooked chicken

- 1/4 teaspoon garlic powder

- 4 cups chicken broth

- 1/2 cup uncooked white rice

- 1/2 cup heavy cream

- Salt and pepper to taste

Instructions:

1. In a large pot over medium heat, melt the butter.

2. Add the onion, celery, and carrots and cook for 5 minutes, stirring occasionally.

3. Add the chicken, garlic powder, and chicken broth and bring to a boil.

4. Reduce heat to low and add the rice. Simmer, covered, for 15 minutes.

5. Add the heavy cream and season with salt and pepper.

6. Simmer for an additional 5 minutes or until the soup is thick and creamy.

Sweet and Sour Pork

Preparation time: 10 minutes, Cooking time: 20 minutes

Ingredients:

- 2 tablespoons vegetable oil

- 1 pound boneless pork, cut into 1-inch cubes

- 1/2 cup diced onion

- 2 cloves garlic, minced

- 1/2 cup diced bell pepper

- 1/4 cup brown sugar

- 1/4 cup white vinegar

- 1/4 cup ketchup

- 1/4 cup pineapple juice

- 1 teaspoon soy sauce

Instructions:

1. Heat the oil in a large skillet over medium heat.

2. Add the pork, onion, garlic, and bell pepper and cook for 5 minutes, stirring occasionally.

3. In a small bowl, mix together the brown sugar, vinegar, ketchup, pineapple juice, and soy sauce.

4. Pour the sauce over the pork and vegetables and stir to combine.

5. Reduce heat to low and simmer for 15 minutes or until the pork is cooked through.

Baked Ziti

Preparation time: 10 minutes, Cooking time: 30 minutes

Ingredients:

- 1 pound ziti pasta

- 1 24-ounce jar of your favorite marinara sauce

- 2 cups ricotta cheese

- 1/2 cup grated Parmesan cheese

- 1 teaspoon garlic powder

- 2 cups shredded mozzarella cheese

- Salt and pepper to taste

Instructions:

1. Preheat oven to 375 degrees F.

2. Cook ziti in boiling salted water for 8 minutes, or until al dente. Drain and set aside.

3. In a medium bowl, combine the marinara sauce, ricotta cheese, Parmesan cheese, garlic powder, salt, and pepper.

4. In a 9x13-inch baking dish, layer half of the cooked ziti, half of the marinara mixture, and half of the mozzarella cheese.

5. Repeat with the remaining ziti, marinara mixture, and mozzarella cheese.

6. Bake in the preheated oven for 20 minutes or until the cheese is melted and bubbly.

Beef and Barley Stew

Preparation time: 10 minutes, Cooking time: 1 hour

Ingredients:

- 2 tablespoons olive oil

- 1 pound stew beef, cubed

- 1/2 cup diced onion

- 1/2 cup diced celery

- 1/2 cup diced carrots

- 4 cups beef broth

- 1/2 cup pearl barley

- 1 teaspoon dried oregano

- 1 teaspoon dried basil

- Salt and pepper to taste

Instructions:

1. Heat the olive oil in a large pot over medium heat.

2. Add the beef, onion, celery, and carrots and cook for 5 minutes, stirring occasionally.

3. Add the beef broth, barley, oregano, and basil. Bring to a boil.

4. Reduce heat to low and simmer, covered, for 45 minutes.

5. Add salt and pepper to taste and simmer for an additional 15 minutes.

Broccoli and Cheddar Quiche

Preparation time: 10 minutes, Cooking time: 45 minutes

Ingredients:

- 1 9-inch unbaked pie crust

- 2 cups chopped fresh broccoli

- 1 cup shredded cheddar cheese

- 4 eggs

- 1 cup milk

- 1/4 teaspoon garlic powder

- Salt and pepper to taste

Instructions:

1. Preheat oven to 350 degrees F.

2. Place the pie crust in a 9-inch pie plate.

3. Sprinkle the broccoli and cheddar cheese into the bottom of the pie crust.

4. In a medium bowl, whisk together the eggs, milk, garlic powder, salt, and pepper.

5. Pour the egg mixture over the broccoli and cheese.

6. Bake in the preheated oven for 45 minutes or until the center is set.

SNACKS

Almond Butter Protein Bites

Introduction: These almond butter protein bites are a great snack for individuals with Alzheimer's or dementia. They're easy to make, satisfying, and full of healthy fats, protein, and fiber.

Ingredients:

- 1 cup almond butter

- ½ cup honey

- ½ cup ground flaxseed

- ½ cup chopped nuts

- ½ cup mini chocolate chips (optional)

- 2 tablespoons chia seeds

- 2 tablespoons hemp hearts

Cooking Instructions:

1. In a medium bowl, mix together the almond butter and honey until smooth.

2. Add the ground flaxseed, chopped nuts, mini chocolate chips (if using), chia seeds, and hemp hearts and mix until everything is evenly distributed.

3. Line a baking sheet with parchment paper and scoop tablespoon-sized portions of the mixture onto the parchment paper.

4. Place in the freezer for 30 minutes to allow the bites to set.

5. Enjoy!

Time: 45 minutes (15 minutes prep, 30 minutes freeze time)

Banana Oat Muffins

Introduction: These banana oat muffins are a great snack for individuals with Alzheimer's or dementia. They're sweet, easy to eat, and full of healthy carbohydrates and fiber.

Ingredients:

- 2 cups rolled oats

- 1 teaspoon baking powder

- ½ teaspoon baking soda

- ½ teaspoon ground cinnamon

- 2 ripe bananas, mashed

- 2 eggs, lightly beaten

- ¼ cup melted coconut oil

- ½ cup honey

- 2 teaspoons vanilla extract

Cooking Instructions:

1. Preheat oven to 350°F.

2. In a medium bowl, mix together the rolled oats, baking powder, baking soda, and cinnamon.

3. In a separate bowl, mix together the mashed bananas, eggs, coconut oil, honey, and vanilla extract.

4. Add the wet ingredients to the dry ingredients and mix until everything is evenly distributed.

5. Grease a muffin tin and scoop the mixture into the muffin cups.

6. Bake for 20 minutes, or until a toothpick inserted into the center of a muffin comes out clean.

7. Enjoy!

Time: 45 minutes (15 minutes prep, 20 minutes bake time)

Trail Mix

Introduction: This trail mix is a great snack for individuals with Alzheimer's or dementia. It's easy to make and full of healthy fats, protein, and fiber.

Ingredients:

- ½ cup raw almonds

- ½ cup raw walnuts

- ½ cup raw cashews

- ½ cup raw pumpkin seeds

- ½ cup dried cranberries

- ½ cup dark chocolate chips

- 2 tablespoons chia seeds

Cooking Instructions:

1. In a medium bowl, mix together the almonds, walnuts, cashews, pumpkin seeds, dried cranberries, dark chocolate chips, and chia seeds.

2. Place in an airtight container and store in the pantry or refrigerator.

3. Enjoy!

Time: 15 minutes (15 minutes prep)

Sweet Potato Fries

Introduction: These sweet potato fries are a great snack for individuals with Alzheimer's or dementia. They're easy to make, satisfying, and full of healthy carbohydrates and fiber.

Ingredients:

- 2 large sweet potatoes, cut into fries

- 2 tablespoons olive oil

- 1 teaspoon garlic powder

- 1 teaspoon dried oregano

- Salt and pepper, to taste

Cooking Instructions:

1. Preheat oven to 400°F.

2. Place the sweet potato fries on a baking sheet and drizzle with olive oil.

3. Sprinkle with garlic powder, oregano, salt, and pepper and mix until everything is evenly distributed.

4. Bake for 20 minutes, flipping the fries halfway through.

5. Enjoy!

Time: 30 minutes (10 minutes prep, 20 minutes bake time)

Avocado Toast

Introduction: Avocado toast is a great snack for individuals with Alzheimer's or dementia. It's simple, quick, and full of healthy fats and fiber.

Ingredients:

- 2 slices of whole wheat bread

- 1 ripe avocado, mashed

- 2 tablespoons olive oil

- Salt and pepper, to taste

Cooking Instructions:

1. Toast the bread slices.

2. In a small bowl, mash the avocado and mix with the olive oil.

3. Spread the avocado mixture on the toast slices and sprinkle with salt and pepper.

4. Enjoy!

Time: 10 minutes (10 minutes prep)

Peanut Butter and Apple Slices

Introduction: Peanut butter and apple slices are a great snack for individuals with Alzheimer's or dementia. They're easy to eat, satisfying, and full of healthy fats and fiber.

Ingredients:

- 2 apples, thinly sliced

- ½ cup peanut butter

- 2 tablespoons honey

Cooking Instructions:

1. Spread the peanut butter on the apple slices.

2. Drizzle with honey.

3. Enjoy!

Time: 5 minutes (5 minutes prep)

Yogurt Parfaits

Introduction: Yogurt parfaits are a great snack for individuals with Alzheimer's or dementia. They're easy to make, satisfying, and full of calcium, protein, and fiber.

Ingredients:

- 2 cups plain Greek yogurt

- ½ cup chopped nuts

- ½ cup dried fruit

- 2 tablespoons honey

Cooking Instructions:

1. In a medium bowl, mix together the Greek yogurt and honey.

2. Layer the yogurt, nuts, and dried fruit in a parfait glass and repeat until the glass is full.

3. Enjoy!

Time: 10 minutes

Kale Chips

Introduction: Kale chips are a great snack for individuals with Alzheimer's or dementia. They're easy to make, satisfying, and full of vitamins, minerals, and fiber.

Ingredients:

- 1 bunch of kale, washed and dried

- 2 tablespoons olive oil

- Salt and pepper, to taste

Cooking Instructions:

1. Preheat oven to 350°F.

2. Place the kale in a large bowl and drizzle with olive oil.

3. Sprinkle with salt and pepper and mix until everything is evenly distributed.

4. Place the kale on a baking sheet and bake for 15 minutes, or until the kale is crispy.

5. Enjoy!

Time: 25 minutes (10 minutes prep, 15 minutes bake time)

Hummus and Veggies

Introduction: Hummus and veggies are a great snack for individuals with Alzheimer's or dementia. They're easy to eat, satisfying, and full of healthy fats, protein, and fiber.

Ingredients:

- 1 cup hummus

- 1 bell pepper, chopped

- 1 cucumber, chopped

- 1 carrot, chopped

- 2 tablespoons olive oil

Cooking Instructions:

1. In a medium bowl, mix together the hummus, bell pepper, cucumber, and carrot.

2. Drizzle with olive oil and mix until everything is evenly distributed.

3. Enjoy!

Time: 15 minutes

Fruit Salad

Introduction: This fruit salad is a great snack for individuals with Alzheimer's or dementia. It's easy to make, satisfying, and full of vitamins, minerals, and fiber.

Ingredients:

- 2 apples, chopped

- 1 banana, chopped

- 1 cup strawberries, chopped

- 1 cup blueberries

- 1 tablespoon honey

Cooking Instructions:

1. In a medium bowl, mix together the apples, banana, strawberries, and blueberries.

2. Drizzle with honey and mix until everything is evenly distributed.

3. Enjoy!

Time: 10 minutes

DESERTS

No-bake Almond Butter Fudge:

Introduction: This delicious no-bake almond butter fudge is a great way to satisfy your sweet tooth without added sugar or dairy.

Ingredients:

¾ cup almond butter

1 tablespoon coconut oil

2 tablespoons maple syrup

½ teaspoon vanilla extract

½ teaspoon ground cinnamon

Pinch of sea salt

Instructions:

1. In a small saucepan, melt together almond butter and coconut oil over low heat.

2. Remove from heat and stir in maple syrup, vanilla extract, cinnamon and sea salt.

3. Line an 8x8 inch baking dish with parchment paper.

4. Pour the almond butter mixture into the dish and spread evenly.

5. Refrigerate for at least 2 hours until set.

6. Cut into small squares and serve.

Cooking Time: 2 hours

Fruit and Nut Bars

Introduction: These delicious fruit and nut bars are full of healthy ingredients and are perfect for a quick snack.

Ingredients:

1 cup dried apricots

1 cup dates

1 cup almonds

1 cup walnuts

1 teaspoon ground cinnamon

1 teaspoon vanilla extract

Instructions:

1. Preheat oven to 350°F.

2. Place the apricots, dates, almonds and walnuts in a food processor and process until a fine crumbly mixture forms.

3. Add the cinnamon and vanilla extract and pulse until combined.

4. Line an 8x8 inch baking dish with parchment paper.

5. Spread the mixture into the dish and press down firmly.

6. Bake for 25 minutes.

7. Let cool before slicing into bars.

Cooking Time: 25 minutes

Chocolate Chip Coconut Cookies

Introduction: These delicious chocolate chip coconut cookies are the perfect treat for a special occasion.

Ingredients:

1 cup coconut oil

1 cup coconut sugar

2 eggs

2 teaspoons vanilla extract

2 ½ cups all-purpose flour

1 teaspoon baking soda

¼ teaspoon salt

2 cups semisweet chocolate chips

Instructions:

1. Preheat oven to 350°F.

2. In a large bowl, cream together coconut oil and coconut sugar until light and fluffy.

3. Add eggs one at a time, beating after each addition.

4. Add vanilla extract and mix until combined.

5. In a separate bowl, combine flour, baking soda and salt.

6. Slowly add the dry ingredients to the wet ingredients and mix until combined.

7. Fold in the chocolate chips.

8. Drop spoonful of the dough onto a baking sheet lined with parchment paper.

9. Bake for 10 minutes.

10. Let cool before serving.

Cooking Time: 10 minutes

Banana Oat Blondies

Introduction: These banana oat blondies are a delicious and healthy alternative to traditional desserts.

Ingredients:

3 ripe bananas, mashed

½ cup coconut oil, melted

1 teaspoon vanilla extract

1 cup rolled oats

¼ teaspoon sea salt

½ cup chopped walnuts

Instructions:

1. Preheat oven to 350°F.

2. In a large bowl, mash the bananas until smooth.

3. Add the melted coconut oil and vanilla extract and mix until combined.

4. Stir in the oats, salt and walnuts.

5. Line an 8x8 inch baking dish with parchment paper.

6. Spread the mixture into the dish and press down firmly.

7. Bake for 25 minutes.

8. Let cool before cutting into bars.

Cooking Time: 25 minutes

Chocolate Pecan Pie

Introduction: This delicious chocolate pecan pie is the perfect dessert for special occasions.

Ingredients:

1 unbaked pie crust

1 cup dark chocolate chips

1 cup light brown sugar

3 eggs

2 tablespoons butter, melted

1 teaspoon vanilla extract

1 cup chopped pecans

Instructions:

1. Preheat oven to 350°F.

2. Place the pie crust in a 9-inch pie dish.

3. Sprinkle the chocolate chips over the crust.

4. In a medium bowl, combine the brown sugar, eggs, butter and vanilla extract.

5. Pour the mixture over the chocolate chips.

6. Sprinkle the chopped pecans over the top.

7. Bake for 45 minutes.

8. Let cool before serving.

Cooking Time: 45 minutes

Strawberry Crumble

Introduction: This delicious strawberry crumble is a perfect summer dessert.

Ingredients:

3 cups fresh strawberries, sliced

1 cup all-purpose flour

½ cup rolled oats

½ cup brown sugar

1 teaspoon ground cinnamon

1 teaspoon ground nutmeg

½ cup melted butter

Instructions:

1. Preheat oven to 350°F.

2. Place the sliced strawberries in an 8x8 inch baking dish.

3. In a medium bowl, combine the flour, oats, brown sugar, cinnamon and nutmeg.

4. Add the melted butter and mix until combined.

5. Sprinkle the mixture over the strawberries.

6. Bake for 30 minutes.

7. Let cool before serving.

Cooking Time: 30 minutes

Chocolate Hazelnut Mousse

Introduction: This light and creamy chocolate hazelnut mousse is the perfect dessert to end a meal.

Ingredients:

3 eggs, separated

¼ cup cocoa powder

¼ cup hazelnut butter

¼ cup honey

1 teaspoon vanilla extract

Instructions:

1. In a medium bowl, beat the egg whites until stiff peaks form.

2. In a separate bowl, beat the egg yolks until light and fluffy.

3. Add the cocoa powder, hazelnut butter, honey and vanilla extract to the egg yolks and mix until combined.

4. Gently fold the egg whites into the egg yolk mixture.

5. Divide the mixture among 4 dessert glasses.

6. Chill in the refrigerator for at least 2 hours.

7. Serve chilled.

Cooking Time: 2 hours

Almond Butter Brownies

Introduction: These delicious almond butter brownies are sure to satisfy any sweet tooth.

Ingredients:

1 cup almond butter

2 eggs

½ cup honey

½ cup cocoa powder

1 teaspoon baking soda

½ teaspoon sea salt

Instructions:

1. Preheat oven to 350°F.

2. In a large bowl, mix together almond butter, eggs and honey until well combined.

3. Add the cocoa powder, baking soda and sea salt and mix until combined.

4. Line an 8x8 inch baking dish with parchment paper.

5. Spread the batter into the dish and bake for 25 minutes.

6. Let cool before slicing into bars.

Cooking Time: 25 minutes

No-bake Almond Coconut Bars

Introduction: These delicious no-bake almond coconut bars are the perfect snack for on-the-go.

Ingredients:

2 cups almond butter

½ cup honey

1 cup shredded coconut

1 cup chopped almonds

1 teaspoon ground cinnamon

Instructions:

1. Line an 8x8 inch baking dish with parchment paper.

2. In a large bowl, mix together almond butter and honey until well combined.

3. Stir in the shredded coconut, chopped almonds and cinnamon.

4. Spread the mixture into the dish and press down firmly.

5. Refrigerate for at least 2 hours until set.

6. Cut into small bars and serve.

Cooking Time: 2 hours

Apple Walnut Crisp

Introduction: This delicious apple walnut crisp is the perfect way to end a meal.

Ingredients:

4 cups apples, peeled and sliced

1 teaspoon ground cinnamon

½ cup chopped walnuts

½ cup all-purpose flour

¼ cup brown sugar

¼ cup melted butter

Instructions:

1. Preheat oven to 350°F.

2. Place the apples in a 9-inch pie dish.

3. Sprinkle the cinnamon over the apples.

4. In a medium bowl, combine the walnuts, flour, brown sugar and melted butter.

5. Sprinkle the mixture over the apples.

6. Bake for 25 minutes.

7. Let cool before serving.

Cooking Time: 25 minutes

SMOOTHIES

Cranberry-Pineapple Smoothie

Introduction: A delicious, fruity smoothie that is packed with antioxidants and vitamins.

Ingredients:

-1/2 cup of frozen cranberries

-1/2 cup of pineapple chunks

-2 tablespoons of honey

-1 cup of plain Greek yogurt

-1/2 cup of milk

-1/2 teaspoon of ground cinnamon

-1/4 teaspoon of ground nutmeg

Cooking Instructions:

1. Place the cranberries, pineapple chunks, honey, yogurt, milk, cinnamon, and nutmeg in a blender.

2. Blend until the mixture is smooth.

3. Pour the mixture into glasses and serve immediately.

Preparation Time: 5 minutes

Acai Berry Smoothie

Introduction: A refreshing smoothie with a fruity flavor that is packed with antioxidants and vitamins.

Ingredients:

-1/2 cup of frozen acai berries

-1/2 cup of frozen blueberries

-1 banana

-2 tablespoons of honey

-1/2 cup of plain Greek yogurt

-1 cup of almond milk

-1/4 teaspoon of ground cinnamon

-1/4 teaspoon of ground nutmeg

Cooking Instructions:

1. Place the acai berries, blueberries, banana, honey, yogurt, almond milk, cinnamon, and nutmeg in a blender.

2. Blend until the mixture is smooth.

3. Pour the mixture into glasses and serve immediately.

Preparation Time: 5 minutes

Blueberry-Mango Smoothie

Introduction: A flavorful smoothie with a tropical twist that is packed with antioxidants and vitamins.

Ingredients:

-1/2 cup of frozen blueberries

-1/2 cup of frozen mango chunks

-2 tablespoons of honey

-1/2 cup of plain Greek yogurt

-1 cup of almond milk

-1/4 teaspoon of ground cinnamon

-1/4 teaspoon of ground nutmeg

Cooking Instructions:

1. Place the blueberries, mango chunks, honey, yogurt, almond milk, cinnamon, and nutmeg in a blender.

2. Blend until the mixture is smooth.

3. Pour the mixture into glasses and serve immediately.

Preparation Time: 5 minutes

Apple-Strawberry Smoothie:

Introduction: A sweet and fruity smoothie that is packed with antioxidants and vitamins.

Ingredients:

-1/2 cup of frozen apples

-1/2 cup of frozen strawberries

-2 tablespoons of honey

-1/2 cup of plain Greek yogurt

-1 cup of almond milk

-1/4 teaspoon of ground cinnamon

-1/4 teaspoon of ground nutmeg

Cooking Instructions:

1. Place the apples, strawberries, honey, yogurt, almond milk, cinnamon, and nutmeg in a blender.

2. Blend until the mixture is smooth.

3. Pour the mixture into glasses and serve immediately.

Preparation Time: 5 minutes

Peach-Raspberry Smoothie

Introduction: A refreshing and vibrant smoothie that is packed with antioxidants and vitamins.

Ingredients:

-1/2 cup of frozen peaches

-1/2 cup of frozen raspberries

-2 tablespoons of honey

-1/2 cup of plain Greek yogurt

-1 cup of almond milk

-1/4 teaspoon of ground cinnamon

-1/4 teaspoon of ground nutmeg

Cooking Instructions:

1. Place the peaches, raspberries, honey, yogurt, almond milk, cinnamon, and nutmeg in a blender.

2. Blend until the mixture is smooth.

3. Pour the mixture into glasses and serve immediately.

Preparation Time: 5 minutes

Pomegranate-Banana Smoothie

Introduction: A creamy and sweet smoothie that is packed with antioxidants and vitamins.

Ingredients:

-1/2 cup of frozen pomegranate seeds

-1 banana

-2 tablespoons of honey

-1/2 cup of plain Greek yogurt

-1 cup of almond milk

-1/4 teaspoon of ground cinnamon

-1/4 teaspoon of ground nutmeg

Cooking Instructions:

1. Place the pomegranate seeds, banana, honey, yogurt, almond milk, cinnamon, and nutmeg in a blender.

2. Blend until the mixture is smooth.

3. Pour the mixture into glasses and serve immediately.

Preparation Time: 5 minutes

Kiwi-Banana Smoothie

Introduction: A sweet and creamy smoothie that is packed with antioxidants and vitamins.

Ingredients:

-1/2 cup of frozen kiwi chunks

-1 banana

-2 tablespoons of honey

-1/2 cup of plain Greek yogurt

-1 cup of almond milk

-1/4 teaspoon of ground cinnamon

-1/4 teaspoon of ground nutmeg

Cooking Instructions:

1. Place the kiwi chunks, banana, honey, yogurt, almond milk, cinnamon, and nutmeg in a blender.

2. Blend until the mixture is smooth.

3. Pour the mixture into glasses and serve immediately.

Preparation Time: 5 minutes

Mango-Orange Smoothie

Introduction: A zesty and fruity smoothie that is packed with antioxidants and vitamins.

Ingredients:

-1/2 cup of frozen mango chunks

-1/2 cup of frozen orange slices

-2 tablespoons of honey

-1/2 cup of plain Greek yogurt

-1 cup of almond milk

-1/4 teaspoon of ground cinnamon

-1/4 teaspoon of ground nutmeg

Cooking Instructions:

1. Place the mango chunks, orange slices, honey, yogurt, almond milk, cinnamon, and nutmeg in a blender.

2. Blend until the mixture is smooth.

3. Pour the mixture into glasses and serve immediately.

Preparation Time: 5 minutes

Pineapple-Banana Smoothie

Introduction: A sweet and creamy smoothie that is packed with antioxidants and vitamins.

Ingredients:

-1/2 cup of frozen pineapple chunks

-1 banana

-2 tablespoons of honey

-1/2 cup of plain Greek yogurt

-1 cup of almond milk

-1/4 teaspoon of ground cinnamon

-1/4 teaspoon of ground nutmeg

Cooking Instructions:

1. Place the pineapple chunks, banana, honey, yogurt, almond milk, cinnamon, and nutmeg in a blender.

2. Blend until the mixture is smooth.

3. Pour the mixture into glasses and serve immediately.

Preparation Time: 5 minutes

Avocado-Blueberry Smoothie:

Introduction: A creamy and nutritious smoothie that is packed with antioxidants and vitamins.

Ingredients:

-1/2 cup of frozen avocado chunks

-1/2 cup of frozen blueberries

-2 tablespoons of honey

-1/2 cup of plain Greek yogurt

-1 cup of almond milk

-1/4 teaspoon of ground cinnamon

-1/4 teaspoon of ground nutmeg

Cooking Instructions:

1. Place the avocado chunks, blueberries, honey, yogurt, almond milk, cinnamon, and nutmeg in a blender.

2. Blend until the mixture is smooth.

3. Pour the mixture into glasses and serve immediately.

Preparation Time: 5 minutes

CONCLUSION

In conclusion, this Alzheimer and Dementia Recipes Cookbook is a great resource for people living with Alzheimer's and Dementia, as well as their caregivers. The recipes are simple, easy to follow, and nutritious. They have been carefully crafted to address the nutritional requirements of those with Alzheimer's and Dementia, as well as to be easy to prepare.

They are also flavorful and easy to modify to suit individual tastes. Furthermore, this cookbook provides a wealth of information about Alzheimer's and Dementia, as well as tips for both those living with Alzheimer's and Dementia, and their caregivers. All in all, this cookbook is an invaluable resource for all those affected by Alzheimer's and Dementia.